GUIDES TO PROSTATE CANCER

Understanding, Managing, and Living Well with Prostate Cancer

Dr. Marvin Charles

Table of Content

CHAPTER 1 4

INTRODUCTION TO PROSTATE CANCER...4

    Diagnosis and Staging 6

    Choices for Treatment 6

    Getting Along with Prostate Cancer....................................7

CHAPTER 2 13

SIGNS AND EARLY FINDING..13

    Ways to Check for Prostate Cancer....................................15

CHAPTER 3 18

DIAGNOSIS OF PROSTATE CANCER 18

CHAPTER 4 20

GRADING AND STAGING 20

    Gleason Score 21

CHAPTER 5 23

TREATMENT PROSTATE CANCER..23

    When to Think About Getting Help.....................................25

    Radiation Therapy 27

CHAPTER 6 30

MANAGING SIDE EFFECTS OF PROSTATE CANCER TREATMENT 30

    Physical Side Effects 31

CHAPTER 7 34

LIVING WITH PROSTATE CANCER..34

CHAPTER 8 37

AFTER TREATMENT AND SURVIVING 37

CHAPTER 9 40

DIET TO IMPROVE CANCER 40

CHAPTER 10 44

HELP AND RESOURCES...44

 CHAPTER 11...47

CONCLUSION...47

CHAPTER 1

INTRODUCTION TO PROSTATE CANCER

Prostate cancer is a common type of cancer that affects many men around the world. Knowing the basics of prostate cancer is important for spotting it early, treating it well, and handling the disease.

What is Prostate Cancer? overgrow Prostate cancer is a disease that happens when cells in the prostate, a small gland in men that helps make semen, start to grow uncontrollably. This can create harmful tumors.

Prostate cancer happens when cells in the prostate gland, a small gland below the bladder and in front of the rectum, start to grow out of control. The prostate is a part of the system that helps men reproduce. It makes a fluid that helps feed and carry sperm.

Different Types of Prostate Cancer.
- Adenocarcinoma: is the predominant type of prostate cancer. It comes from the gland cells in the prostate gland.

- Small Cell Carcinomas: A rare and fast-growing type of cancer.

- Neuroendocrine tumors are rare and usually overgrow.

- Transitional Cell Carcinomas start in the urethra cells and can spread to the prostate.

Things That Might Cause Problems
- Age: The risk goes up a lot after you turn 50.

- Family History: If someone in your family had prostate cancer, your risk of getting it is twice as high.

- Race: African American men have a higher risk than men from other races.

- Genetics: Some gene changes you get from your parents can make you more likely to have a certain risk.

- Lifestyle: How we eat, our weight, and not exercising can affect our health risks.
Signs of a problem or illness.

In the beginning, prostate cancer usually doesn't show any clear signs. As cancer gets worse, you might start to see these signs:

Trouble urinating
- Slow or disrupted urine flow
Going to the bathroom often, especially during the night.

- Pain or burning when you pee

- Blood in urine or semen means seeing blood when you pee or in your sperm.

- Painful ejaculation means having discomfort or pain when ejaculating.

- Constant pain in the back, hips, or lower stomach area.
Screening and Detection

Finding prostate cancer early can greatly help in getting better treatment results.

Some common ways to check for things are:
- Prostate-Specific Antigen (PSA) Test: Checks how much PSA is in the blood. High levels might mean there is prostate cancer.

- Digital Rectal Exam (DRE): A doctor checks the prostate by feeling it with a gloved finger.

Diagnosis and Staging

If the screening tests show signs of prostate cancer, more tests will be done to check for it.

Biopsy: A piece of prostate tissue is looked at under a microscope.

Imaging Tests: MRI, CT scans, and bone scans are used to see how far the cancer has spread.

The stage of prostate cancer depends on how big the tumor is, whether the lymph nodes are affected, and if the cancer has spread to other places. The stages go from I (early) to IV (advanced).

Choices for Treatment

The treatment for prostate cancer depends on how advanced the cancer is, the patient's general health, and what the patient prefers.

Here are some choices:

Active Surveillance: Keeping a close watch on the cancer without treating it right away.

Surgery: Taking out the prostate gland (radical prostatectomy).

Radiation Therapy: Using strong rays to destroy cancer cells.

Hormone Therapy: Lowering the amount of male hormones that help cancer grow.

Chemotherapy: Using medicine to kill cancer cells.

Immunotherapy: Strengthening the body's defense system to help fight cancer.

Targeted Therapy: Medications that focus on certain functions of cancer cells.

Clinical Trials: Getting new and experimental treatments.

Getting Along with Prostate Cancer

Living with prostate cancer means dealing with both physical and emotional difficulties. Help from doctors, family, and support groups is very important. Patients are urged to keep a healthy lifestyle, learn about their health condition, and take part in their treatment.

Outlook or expected outcome.

The outlook for prostate cancer depends on how advanced it is when it's found and how well the treatment works. Early-stage prostate cancer has a good chance of survival, but advanced-stage cancer needs more serious treatment and care.

Knowing about prostate cancer helps patients and their families make better choices about treatment and enhance their quality of life.

Causes and Risk Factors
Prostate cancer happens when cells in the prostate gland start to grow too much and out of control. We don't know the exact reason why prostate cancer happens, but some things might make a man more likely to get it. These factors include genes, ways of living, and surroundings.

Genetic Factors
Genes have a big impact on the chances of getting prostate cancer. Most prostate cancer cases happen by chance, but a significant number are linked to genetics. It's important to know how genes affect health so we can find people who are more at risk and create tailored plans for prevention and treatment.

Family Background
Family-linked Prostate Cancer
About 5-10% of prostate cancer cases run in families.

Men who have a close family member, like a father or brother, with prostate cancer are twice as likely to get the disease themselves.

The risk goes up even more if many family members are affected or if a relative got diagnosed when they were young.

Family Grouping
The fact that prostate cancer often runs in families indicates that there may be a genetic link. Men who have many family members with certain health problems are more likely to have those problems themselves.

Inherited Genetic Changes
BRCA1 and BRCA2 are genes in our bodies. They help repair damaged DNA. If there are problems with these genes, it can increase the risk of certain cancers, especially breast and ovarian cancer.

Changes in the BRCA1 and BRCA2 genes, which are often linked to breast and ovarian cancers, can also raise the chance of getting prostate cancer.

Men with BRCA2 mutations have a greater risk of getting prostate cancer than those with BRCA1 mutations, and they are more likely to develop serious types of the disease.

HOXB13 is a gene.
The HOXB13 gene change (G84E) is connected to a higher chance of developing prostate cancer at a younger age.
This mutation is uncommon, but it greatly increases the risk for those who carry it.

Genes that help fix DNA

Changes in certain genes that help fix DNA, like ATM, CHEK2, and PALB2, can raise the chances of getting prostate cancer.
These changes can make DNA unstable, which can cause cancer to grow.

Genetic Variations
Single Nucleotide Polymorphisms (SNPs) are small differences in the DNA sequence that occur when one building block (nucleotide) is replaced by another.

Studies looking at the entire genome have found many genetic changes (SNPs) that are linked to the risk of prostate cancer.

Each SNP adds a little to the chances of risk, but together, they can affect how likely someone is to be at risk.
Commonly studied SNPs are found in areas like 8q24, where several variations can increase the risk of prostate cancer.

Polygenic Risk Scores are a way to estimate a person's chance of developing certain traits or diseases based on the combined effects of many genes.

Polygenic risk scores add together the effects of many small genetic differences to estimate how likely someone is to get prostate cancer.

These scores can help find people who are at high risk and might need more tests and preventive care.

Differences in Ethnic and Racial Groups
African Roots

Men with African heritage are more likely to get prostate cancer than men from other ethnic groups.

Genetic studies have found some gene variations that are more common in African populations, which add to the higher risk.

European and Asian Backgrounds
Genetic differences linked to the risk of prostate cancer also change between men of European and Asian backgrounds.

It's important to understand these differences to create screening and prevention plans that work for specific groups of people.

Genetic Counseling and Testing means getting advice and information about your genes. It helps you understand if you might pass on certain health problems to your kids and if testing for these problems might be helpful.

Rules for Genetic Testing
Men who have a strong family background of prostate cancer, especially if it started early or if many family members are affected, might find it helpful to talk to a genetic counselor and get tested.
Testing for the BRCA1, BRCA2, and other important genes can help assess and manage risk effectively.

Effects of Genetic Testing
Positive test results for risky mutations can help make choices about check-ups, screenings, and prevention actions.

Genetic information can affect treatment decisions, like using PARP inhibitors for patients with BRCA mutations.

Studying and What's Next
Current Research
Ongoing studies are looking for more genetic reasons that might increase the risk of prostate cancer.
Understanding how genes and the environment work together is important for evaluating risks fully.
Precision Medicine refers to a way of treating illnesses that takes into account a person's unique characteristics, like their genes, environment, and lifestyle. This approach helps doctors create personalized treatments that are more effective for each individual.

Discoveries in genetics are helping us create precision medicine. This means using people's genetic information to tailor prevention, screening, and treatment plans just for them.
Treatments aimed at specific genetic changes show potential for helping prostate cancer patients do better.

Ways of Living and Environmental Impact

Knowing how our lifestyle and surroundings can affect us can help lower the chances of getting prostate cancer. Here are some main ideas explained in easy words:

Food Plan

Red and Processed Meats

Eating a lot of red meat (like beef and pork) and processed meats (like bacon and sausages) might raise the chance of getting prostate cancer.

High-Fat Dairy Foods

Eating a lot of high-fat dairy foods, like cheese and butter, could increase the risk.

Fruits and Vegetables

Eating a lot of fruits and vegetables can help reduce the chances of getting sick. They have vitamins and nutrients that are good for your body.

How Much Calcium You Should Eat

Too much calcium, especially from supplements, can be harmful even though calcium is good for bones.

Obesity means having a lot of extra weight. It happens when a person has more body fat than is healthy.

Body Weight.

Being very overweight can raise the chances of getting prostate cancer. Maintaining a healthy weight by eating well and being active can lower this risk.

Exercise

Move your body to stay healthy.
Regular exercise may help reduce the chances of getting prostate cancer. It also supports general health and can help keep a healthy weight.

Using Tobacco
Smoking doesn't directly cause prostate cancer, but it can raise the chances of getting more severe forms of the disease and lead to worse outcomes.

Drinking Alcohol:
Drinking a lot of alcohol can raise the chance of getting prostate cancer. It's a good idea to drink a little or not at all.

Age and Race
Age
The chance of getting prostate cancer increases as men get older, especially after they turn 50.

Ethnicity refers to a group of people who share common characteristics such as culture, language, and traditions.

African American men are more likely to get prostate cancer and often get it at an earlier age than men from other ethnic groups.

Asian and Hispanic men usually have lower risks.

Hormonal Factors
Testosterone is a hormone that helps develop male traits and maintain health in both men and women.
Higher amounts of testosterone, which is a male hormone, can raise the chance of getting prostate cancer. This hormone helps prostate cancer cells get bigger.

Swelling and Infections
Prostate Swelling
Long-term swelling of the prostate (called prostatitis) and certain infections may raise the chance of getting prostate cancer.
Chemical Exposure means coming into contact with harmful chemicals.

Harmful substances and chemicals
Being around certain chemicals, like those in pesticides or used in some workplaces, might raise the chance of getting prostate cancer.

Vasectomy is a medical procedure that makes a man unable to father children.

It means cutting and closing the tubes that carry sperm from the testicles.

Surgery History

Some studies say that there might be a slight increase in risk after a vasectomy (which is a surgery to stop sperm from being released), but the evidence is not definite.

CHAPTER 2

SIGNS AND EARLY FINDING

It's important to know the signs of prostate cancer and how to catch it early for better treatment and results. Below are easy ways to explain it:

Common Signs

Prostate cancer usually doesn't show any signs when it first starts, but as it gets worse, some symptoms might start to show.

Below are the signs to look out for:

Problems with Urinating

- Trouble starting to pee or stopping once you've started.
- A slow or interrupted stream of urine.
-Feeling to urinate more often, especially during the night.
-Feeling like your bladder is still full even after you have gone to the bathroom.

Soreness or Unease

- Discomfort or a burning feeling when you pee.
- Painful ejaculation. Rewritten: - Hurting when you ejaculate.
-Ongoing pain in the lower back, hips, or pelvic area.

Blood

-Blood in your pee.
-Blood in your sperm.
-Problems with getting or keeping an erection.

- Trouble getting or keeping an erection.

The Importance of Finding Problems Early

Finding prostate cancer early is important for better treatment and results. Here is why finding problems early is really important:

Improved Treatment Choices

When prostate cancer is detected early, there are more ways to treat it. These can be milder and cause fewer problems.

Better chances of surviving

Prostate cancer that is found early has a much better chance of survival than cancer that has spread to other areas of the body. Almost all men with early-stage prostate cancer live for at least five years after they are diagnosed.

Gentler Treatment

Finding cancer early can allow for treatments that are easier on the body, like just watching the cancer closely instead of starting treatment right away. This can help prevent or postpone the side effects of tougher treatments like surgery or radiation.

Better Living Conditions

Finding and treating prostate cancer early can help lower the chances of problems like losing control over urination or having trouble with erections.

This can make life better.

Calm Feeling

Regular check-ups and being aware of your health can make you feel more at ease. If cancer is found, it can be treated quickly.

Affordable

Finding and treating cancer early can save money compared to treating cancer that has progressed, which often needs more complicated and longer treatments.

Ways to Find Out Early

-PSA Test (Prostate-Specific Antigen Test)

-A blood test that checks how much PSA, a protein made by the prostate, is in your blood. High levels may be an early sign of prostate cancer.

-Digital Rectal Exam (DRE) is a medical test where a doctor checks the inside of your rectum using their finger. This exam helps them find any problems in the prostate or other areas.
A doctor checks the prostate gland by feeling it through the rectum to look for any problems or lumps.

Who Needs to Be Tested?
Men over the age of 50
Men over 50 should talk to their doctor about tests for prostate cancer.

Groups with Higher Risk
Men who are at greater risk, like African American men or those who have family members with prostate cancer, should think about starting tests earlier, around age 45 or even younger.40.

Ways to Check for Prostate Cancer
Testing for prostate cancer helps find the disease early, which improves the chances of successful treatment. The two most common tests for checking prostate health are the PSA test and the Digital Rectal Exam (DRE).

-PSA Test (Prostate-Specific Antigen Test)
What is the PSA Test?
The PSA test is a blood test that checks how much prostate-specific antigen (PSA) is in your blood. PSA is a protein made by the prostate gland, and higher amounts of it can suggest the presence of prostate cancer.

How is the PSA Test Performed?
A doctor takes a sample of your blood and sends it to a lab to check the PSA level.
What Do PSA Levels Mean?
Normal PSA levels are usually 4. 0 ng/mL or less, but what counts as "normal" can be different for each person.

-High PSA levels: If your PSA levels are higher than normal, it could mean you have prostate cancer. However, it can also be caused by other things like an enlarged prostate or inflammation of the prostate.

Benefits of PSA Testing
-Can find prostate cancer early, often before signs show up.
- Easy and safe blood test.

Drawbacks of PSA Testing

High PSA levels don't always mean there is cancer, which can lead to false alarms.

Some prostate cancers don't make a lot of PSA, which can result in missing a diagnosis.

This can cause extra worry and lead to more tests or treatments that aren't needed.

Digital Rectal Exam (DRE)

What is a Digital Rectal Exam (DRE)?

The DRE is a check-up where a doctor feels the prostate gland for any problems by putting a finger in the rectum.

How is the DRE Performed?

During the exam, the doctor wears a glove and uses a lubricated finger to check the size, shape, and feel of the prostate inside the rectum.

What Can the DRE Find.?

Unusual bumps, hard spots, or strange shapes could mean cancer.

Benefits of the DRE

Can find problems in the prostate that might not be seen in a PSA test.

A quick and easy process that can be done during a regular health check-up.

Drawbacks of the DRE

Not as good at finding early prostate cancer as the PSA test.

It might overlook tumors that are not close to the rectal wall.

Using PSA and DRE together

Better Detection

Using both PSA tests and DRE exams together can help find prostate cancer early.

If the results from either test are not normal, doctors usually recommend more tests, like a prostate biopsy.

Who Should Be Checked?

Men Who Are 50 and Older

Men are usually told to begin talking to their doctor about prostate cancer tests when they turn 50.

Groups at High Risk

Men who are more likely to get prostate cancer, like African American men or those with family members who had it, should think about getting screened earlier, around age 45 or even 40.

CHAPTER 3

DIAGNOSIS OF PROSTATE CANCER

If screening tests like the PSA test or DRE show that there might be prostate cancer, more tests are needed to confirm if the cancer is there and to find out how far it has spread. Here's a simple explanation of the diagnostic process:

First Steps
-Health History and Physical Checkup
Your doctor will look at your medical records and do a physical check-up, including a special exam, to see if there are any problems with your prostate.

-PSA Test (Prostate-Specific Antigen Test)
If it wasn't done during the screening, a PSA test might be done again to check if the levels are high and to see how they change over time.

-Tests that help find out if something is wrong.
Transrectal Ultrasound (TRUS) is a test that uses sound waves to create pictures of the prostate gland. It involves placing a small device into the rectum to get clear images.

A small device is placed in the rectum to take pictures of the prostate using

sound waves. TRUS can help spot unusual areas and direct biopsy needles.
Prostate Biopsy: A test to take a small sample of tissue from the prostate gland to check for problems or cancer.

A biopsy is the best way to find out if someone has prostate cancer. During the procedure, tiny pieces of prostate tissue are collected and looked at under a microscope to check for cancer cells.

Transrectal Biopsy: This is the most usual way to take a sample, where needles go in through the rectum.
Transperineal Biopsy: Needles are put through the skin between the anus and the scrotum. This method is sometimes used when the transrectal method cannot be used.

Testing with Images

Magnetic Resonance Imaging (MRI) is a medical test that uses magnets and radio waves to take detailed pictures of the inside of your body.

An MRI gives clear pictures of the prostate and the areas nearby. It can help check how much cancer there is and point to specific parts of the prostate for taking samples.
MRI Fusion Biopsy: Uses pictures from MRI and ultrasound to accurately find and target areas of concern during a biopsy.

-Bone Scan
If there's a chance that cancer has moved to the bones, a doctor might do a bone scan. It means putting a tiny bit of radioactive material into the body and using a special camera to find any unusual spots.

-CT Scan (Computed Tomography Scan)
A CT scan takes clear pictures of slices of the body to see if cancer has spread to other organs.

-PET Scan (Positron Emission Tomography)
A PET scan uses a special substance that has mild radioactivity to find cancer cells. Sometimes, it is used together with a CT scan to get clearer pictures.

CHAPTER 4

GRADING AND STAGING

Gleason Score

The Gleason score measures how similar prostate cancer cells are to normal prostate cells when looked at under a microscope. Scores go from 6 (not very aggressive) to 10 (very aggressive).

TNM Staging System is a way to describe how cancer is growing in the body. It looks at three main things: - **T** tells how big the tumor is and if it's spread to nearby areas. - **N** shows if cancer has spread close to lymph nodes. - **M** indicates if cancer has spread to other parts of the body. This system helps doctors understand the stage of cancer and decide on the best treatment.

The TNM system ranks cancer according to:
T (Tumor): The size and spread of the main tumor.

N (Nodes): This tells us if cancer has spread to nearby lymph nodes.
M (Metastasis): If cancer has moved to other areas of the body.

Types of Risks
Prostate cancer is usually grouped into risk levels (low, medium, high) based on PSA test results, Gleason score, and the TNM stage. This helps doctors decide on treatment.

Genetic and DNA Testing
Genetic Testing
Genetic tests can find certain changes in genes that may affect treatment choices and give details about the chance of having a serious type of cancer.

Genomic tests look at how genes work in cancer cells to help understand how the cancer might act and how it will respond to treatment.

Understanding the Levels and Types of Prostate Cancer
Knowing the stage and grade of prostate cancer is important for figuring out the best treatments and for predicting what will happen next.

Here's an easy way to explain staging and grading:
Grading: The Gleason Score
What is the Gleason Score?
The Gleason score checks how similar prostate cancer cells are to healthy cells when looked at under a microscope. It helps show how fast the cancer will grow and spread.

How is the Gleason Score decided?
Two parts of the prostate that have the most cancer are looked at, and each one is given a score from 3 to 5.
The two scores are added together to make a Gleason score that ranges from 6 to 10.

What Do the Scores Mean?
Gleason 6 (3+3): A type of cancer that is not aggressive. The cells look quite like normal cells and probably grow slowly.

Gleason 7 (3+4 or 4+3): A type of cancer that is in the middle range of seriousness. The cells are more unusual and might grow at a steady speed.

Gleason 8-10 (4+4, 4+5, or 5+5): This means it's a type of aggressive cancer. The cells look unusual compared to regular cells and are probably going to grow fast

Types of Risks

By looking at the Gleason score, TNM stages, and PSA levels together, we can sort prostate cancer into different risk groups. This helps doctors figure out the best treatment plan.
Low Risk.
PSA is lower than 10 ng/mL.
Gleason score of 6 or less.
Cancer that is only in the prostate (T1-T2a).

Intermediate Risk

PSA levels are between 10 and 20 ng/mL.
Gleason score of 7.
Cancer that is only in the prostate (T2b-T2c).
High Risk means there is a big chance of something bad happening.
PSA higher than 20 ng/mL.
Gleason score of 8 to 10.
Cancer has spread beyond the prostate.

CHAPTER 5

TREATMENT PROSTATE CANCER

Treatment for prostate cancer relies on a few important things: how advanced the cancer is, how serious it is, the patient's general health, and what the patient prefers. Here are the main ways to treat it:

Watching Prostate Cancer Closely

Active surveillance is a way to manage prostate cancer by watching the condition carefully without starting treatment right away. This method is usually suggested for men who have low-risk, slow-growing prostate cancer. Here's a summary:

What is Active Surveillance? Active Surveillance is a way to closely monitor a person's health condition, usually for diseases like cancer, without starting immediate treatment. Instead of treating right away, doctors watch for any changes over time to decide the best next steps.

Active surveillance means keeping a close watch on prostate cancer by doing different tests and check-ups to see if there are any changes in the cancer. The aim is to prevent or postpone treatments like surgery or radiation, which can cause serious side effects, while still managing the cancer effectively.

Who is a Good Fit for Watching and Waiting?

Low-Risk Prostate Cancer
Gleason score of 6 or less.
PSA level is below 10 ng/mL.
Cancer that is only in the prostate gland and hasn't spread (stages T1 to T2a).
Other Things

Men who are likely to live longer and are still suitable for future treatments if necessary.
Men who want to skip or put off possible side effects of treatment, like trouble with urinating and having sex.

Watching Plan
Active surveillance means having regular tests and check-ups to keep an eye on how prostate cancer is developing. These usually include:
Prostate-Specific Antigen (PSA) Test: A blood test that checks for a substance made by the prostate gland. It helps find problems like prostate cancer.
Regular blood tests to check PSA levels.

- How often: Usually every 3 to 6 months.

Digital Rectal Exam (DRE) is a medical test where a doctor checks the health of your lower abdomen and rectum by inserting a gloved finger into the rectum.

Physical check-ups to look for changes in the prostate.
- How often: Usually every 6 to 12 months.

Prostate Biopsy A prostate biopsy is a medical test where a doctor takes small samples of tissue from the prostate gland to check for cancer or other problems.

Regular tissue samples to check the cancer's Gleason score and stage.
- Frequency: Typically every 1 to 3 years, or more often if there are changes in PSA levels or results from a digital rectal exam (DRE).

Magnetic Resonance Imaging (MRI) is a medical test that uses magnets and radio waves to take detailed pictures of the inside of the body.

MRIs can take clear pictures of the prostate and help find any problem areas.

- Frequency: As the doctor suggested, it's usually used before biopsies to help with the sampling.

When to Think About Getting Help

If you are being watched closely for cancer and it shows signs of getting worse, your doctor might suggest starting treatment. Reasons for treatment include:

Increasing PSA Levels
A steady and noticeable rise in PSA levels over time.

Changes in DRE can be simplified to: "Updates in DRE.
New lumps or hard spots in the prostate.
Test Results from a Biopsy
A higher Gleason score or signs that the cancer is spreading.

MRI Results
New or increased problems were found on the MRI.
Advantages of Watching Closely

Avoidance of Side Effects.

It helps avoid or postpone possible problems from treatments like surgery or radiation, such as trouble with urination, erectile issues, and bowel problems.

Maintaining Quality of Life

Let men keep living their usual lives and doing their daily activities without feeling the immediate effects of cancer treatments.

Less Invasive

It means watching closely instead of doing quick, uncomfortable treatments.

Potential Risks and Challenges

-Cancer Progression
There is a chance that the cancer might grow or become more serious while being watched.

-Anxiety and Stress
Not knowing what will happen when you have cancer that isn't being treated can make you feel very stressed and upset.

Need Regular Check-Ups

Having tests and exams often can be stressful and hard for some patients.

Surgery: Radical Prostatectomy
What is Radical Prostatectomy
Radical Prostatectomy is a surgery to remove the prostate gland and some close tissue from a man's body.

Types of Radical Prostate Surgery:

-Open Radical Prostatectomy: A surgery to remove the prostate gland and some surrounding tissue through a large cut in the abdomen.

-Laparoscopic Radical Prostatectomy
Minimally invasive surgery uses small cuts and a camera.

- Robot-Aided Laparoscopic Surgery for Prostate Removal:
It's like regular laparoscopic surgery, but it uses robots to help make it more precise.

Advantages:
It might be possible to get rid of the cancer if it is only in the prostate.
- Gives a clear report about the disease.

Risks and Possible Problems:
-Urinary incontinence.

-Erectile dysfunction .
There is a chance of problems like infections or losing too much blood.

Radiation Therapy

What is Radiation Therapy? Radiation therapy is a treatment that uses high-energy rays, similar to X-rays, to kill cancer cells. It helps shrink tumors and can be used alone or with other treatments like surgery or chemotherapy.
Uses strong beams of energy or particles to destroy cancer cells.

Types of Radiation Treatment:

External Beam Radiation Therapy (EBRT) is a treatment that uses high-energy rays to kill cancer cells. These rays come from a machine outside the body and are directed at the area with cancer.

Radiation is aimed at the prostate from outside the body.

Brachytherapy: This is a type of treatment where doctors place small radioactive seeds inside or near a tumor to help kill cancer cells.
It means putting small radioactive seeds straight into the prostate.

Advantages:
- Not requiring surgery (for EBRT).
-It can be a choice for people who aren't good candidates for surgery.

Risks and Problems:
- Tiredness.
- Problems with peeing (needing to go often, feeling a strong need to go, leaking).
- Problems with the bowels (like diarrhea or bleeding from the bottom).
-Erectile dysfunction means having trouble getting or keeping an erection.
-Hormone Treatment (Androgen Deprivation Treatment - ADT)

What is Hormone Therapy?
It lowers the amount of male hormones to prevent them from helping prostate cancer cells grow.

Types of Hormone Treatment:
-LHRH Agonists and Antagonists: LHRH agonists are drugs that help to increase the levels of certain hormones in the body, while LHRH antagonists are drugs that block those hormones.
Medications that reduce testosterone levels.

- Anti-Androgens:
Stop the effect of testosterone.

- Orchiectomy: This is a surgery to remove one or both testicles.
Surgery to take out the testicles to lower testosterone levels.

Advantages:
-It slows the growth of prostate cancer.
- Can make tumors smaller before other treatments.

Dangers and Unwanted Effects:
-Hot flashes are sudden feelings of warmth that can make you feel really hot and sometimes sweaty.
-Loss of interest in sex and trouble getting or keeping an erection.

- Weak bones (osteoporosis).
-Tiredness and gaining weight.

What is Chemotherapy? Chemotherapy is a cancer treatment. It uses strong medicines to kill cancer cells or stop them from growing. These medicines can be given as pills or through a needle in your arm.
Uses medicine to destroy fast-growing cancer cells, usually given through a vein or taken by mouth.

When is Chemotherapy Used?
Advanced prostate cancer that has spread to other areas of the body.
When hormone treatment stops working.

Common Cancer Medicines:
Docetaxel is a type of medicine used to treat some kinds of cancer.
Cabazitaxel is a medicine used to treat certain types of cancer.

Advantages:
-It can lessen symptoms and help people live longer in serious cases.
-Dangers and Unwanted Effects:
- Losing hair.
-Feeling sick to your stomach and throwing up.
-Higher chance of getting infections.
-Tiredness

Immunotherapy

Immunotherapy is a type of treatment that helps the body's immune system fight diseases, especially cancer.
• Uses the body's defense system to battle cancer.

Types of Immunotherapy:
-Sipuleucel-T (also known as Provenge) is a type of cancer treatment.
A cancer vaccine that helps the immune system fight prostate cancer cells.
-Immune Checkpoint Blockers:
-Medicines that assist the immune system in spotting and fighting cancer cells.

Advantages:
It can work well for severe prostate cancer.
Usually easy to get along with.
Dangers and Unwanted Effects:

Cold-like symptoms.

Targeted Therapy
Targeted Therapy uses drugs to focus on certain molecules that contribute to cancer growth and spreading.

Types of Targeted Treatment:
-PARP Inhibitors:
Examples include olaparib and rucaparib, which are used to treat prostate cancer with certain gene changes (BRCA1/2).

Advantages:
It hits cancer cells more accurately, which means it doesn't hurt normal cells as much.
Dangers and Possible Problems:
-Feeling sick to your stomach.
-Tiredness
-Anemia

Clinical Trials are tests done to find out if new medicines or treatments work and are safe for people.

Advantages:
-Access to the latest treatments.
-Helping with medical research.
-Things to think about:
-Possible unknown dangers and side effects.
-Not all patients may qualify.

CHAPTER 6

MANAGING SIDE EFFECTS OF PROSTATE CANCER TREATMENT

Treatments for prostate cancer can cause different side effects that may affect a person's physical health, emotions, and mental state.

Here are simple guide on how to handle these side effects:

Physical Side Effects

Incontinence

Types of Incontinence:

-Stress Incontinence: Leaking urine when doing things that pressure your belly, like coughing or lifting heavy things.

-Urge Incontinence: A sudden, strong feeling that you need to pee, which can lead to leaking urine without being able to control it.

Ways to Manage:

-Pelvic Floor Exercises (Kegels): Strengthening the muscles that help control when you pee.

-Bladder Training: Going to the bathroom at set times and slowly waiting longer in-between visits.

-Medicines: Pills that help calm bladder cramps.

-Surgery: Treatments like using special slings or fake sphincters for serious cases.
-Erectile Dysfunction (ED).

Causes:
-Nerve injury from surgery or radiation.
-Less blood is going to the penis.
-Management Strategies: Simple Ways to Lead and Organize a Team.
-Medications: Pills like sildenafil (Viagra), tadalafil (Cialis), and vardenafil (Levitra).
-Vacuum Erection Devices: Machines that help create erections.
-Penile Injections: Medicine put directly into the penis.
-Penile implants: Surgery options for very serious cases.
-Counseling: Support for feeling anxious and stressed because of eating problems.

Anxiety and Depression
Ways to Manage:
Counseling and Therapy: Talking to a mental health expert, either alone or in a group.
- Support Groups: Meeting with other people who have prostate cancer to help each other.
- Medicines: You might need antidepressants or medications for anxiety.

Body Image and Self-Worth
Ways to Manage:
- Talk openly: Share your worries with a partner or a counselor.
Mindfulness and Relaxation Techniques: Ways to calm down and feel less stressed, like meditating and doing yoga.
- Good Lifestyle Changes: Doing things that make you feel more confident and happy.

Food Choices to Think About
Diet and Prostate Cancer
Recommended Diet:
-Fruits and vegetables are full of vitamins, minerals, and helpful substances.
-Whole Grains: Good sources of fiber and vitamins.
- Lean Proteins: These include fish, chicken, beans, and other similar foods.
- Good Fats: Eat omega-3 fats found in fish and flaxseeds.

Foods to Eat Less Of:
Red and processed meats: Linked to a higher chance of getting cancer.
High-fat dairy products might increase the risk of prostate cancer.
Sugary foods and drinks have few nutrients and can make you gain weight.

Hydration
Drink enough water: It is important to stay hydrated for your overall health
and to help you recover.

Vitamins and extra nutrients
Talk to a doctor: Some supplements might affect cancer treatments or
prostate health.

Physical Therapy and Recovery
-Pelvic Floor Physical Therapy: This is a type of exercise and treatment that
helps strengthen the muscles in the lower part of your stomach and pelvis. It
can help with issues like pain, incontinence, and discomfort during sex.

-Kegel Exercises: These exercises help make the pelvic floor muscles stronger
and improve control over the bladder.

-Biofeedback: This helps keep track of and improve how you control your
muscles.
Regular Physical Therapy

Goals:
Get Stronger and Move Better: Simple exercises to help you function well
physically.
- Handle Pain: Ways to lessen pain after treatment.
- Improve Quality of Life: Actions that support good health and happiness.

Exercise Plans
Benefits:
- Better Physical Health: Less tiredness, stronger heart, and helps with keeping
a healthy weight.
- Mental Health Benefits: Helps reduce feelings of worry and sadness, and
improves your mood.

Types of Exercise:
-Aerobic Exercise: Moving activities like walking, swimming, and riding a bike.

-Strength Training: Using weights and resistance bands to build muscles.
Flexibility Exercises: Stretching and yoga.

CHAPTER 7

LIVING WITH PROSTATE CANCER

Having prostate cancer can lead to many big changes and difficulties, both in your body and feelings.

Here are some ways and tools to help deal with these changes and keep a good life.

Coping Strategies

Keep Updated

Learn about prostate cancer, how it can be treated, and the possible side effects.
Keep informed about the newest studies and updates.

Keep Talking Openly

Talk about your feelings, worries, and concerns with your doctors, family, and friends.
Feel free to ask questions or share what you need.

Set Achievable Goals

Focus on things you can change and make goals that are easy to reach.
Celebrate little wins and steps forward.

Practice being present and calming yourself.
Try doing things like meditation, deep breathing, or yoga to help lower stress and worry.
Think about using methods like tensing and relaxing your muscles or imagining peaceful scenes.

Keep moving
Make sure to include regular exercise in your daily life, based on what you can do and how much energy you have.
Activities like walking, swimming, and light weight lifting can make you healthier in both body and mind.

Counseling
Join prostate cancer support groups to talk about your experiences, learn new things, and get support.
Support groups, whether they meet in person or online, can be helpful.

Peer Support Programs
Talking one-on-one with a therapist or counselor can help you deal with feelings of anxiety, depression, and other emotional problems.
Family counseling can help your family talk and understand each other better.

Programs for Helping Each Other
Programs that help you meet people with similar experiences can offer helpful tips and emotional help.
Community Resources are the services and help available to people in the community.
Find local groups and cancer support centers that provide classes, workshops, and social events.

Lifestyle Changes
Eating Healthy
-Eat a healthy diet that includes plenty of fruits, vegetables, whole grains, and lean meats.
-Reduce how much red meat, processed meat, fatty dairy foods, and sugary snacks and drinks you eat.

Working Out Regularly
Try to do at least 150 minutes of moderate exercise or 75 minutes of intense exercise every week, and also include some strength training exercises.

Change your workout plan according to how you feel and what your body can do.

Getting Enough Rest
Make sure you get enough sleep and rest so your body can heal and handle tiredness better.
Make sure to go to bed wake up at the same time every day, and create a cozy place to sleep.

Stay away from tobacco and drink less alcohol.
Stop smoking and steer clear of tobacco products.
Keep drinking alcohol to a moderate amount.

Sexual Health and Close Relationships
Talk Openly with Your Partner
Talk to your partner about your feelings, worries, and any changes in your sexual ability.
Work together to discover new ways to keep your connection strong and close.

Get Help from a Professional
Think about visiting a therapist or counselor who knows about sexual health and intimacy problems that can come up because of cancer.
Talk to your doctor about possible ways to treat erectile dysfunction or other sexual problems.

Use available treatments.
Medicines like Viagra or Cialis, and devices like vacuum pumps, can help treat erectile dysfunction.
Penile implants or injections might be choices for some men.
Look into different ways to feel close to people.
Focus on ways to be close without having sex, like hugging, kissing, and gentle touching.
Talk honestly about what feels nice and satisfying for both people.

CHAPTER 8

AFTER TREATMENT AND SURVIVING

After treatment for prostate cancer, it's important to focus on healing and staying healthy for the future. Survivorship means taking care of people after they have had cancer. This includes checking for any signs of cancer coming back, helping with long-term health problems, and making sure they have a good quality of life.

Follow-Up Care
Regular: Health Checkups
Frequency Usually every 3 to 6 months for the first few years, then less often if there are no problems.

Parts: Check-ups, PSA tests, and maybe pictures (like scans) if necessary. Prostate-specific antigen (PSA) Tests are blood tests used to check for a substance made by the prostate gland that can help identify prostate issues.

Regular PSA tests help check for any signs that cancer might come back.
-Schedule: Usually every 3 to 6 months at first, then once a year if PSA levels stay the same.

Digital Rectal Exam (DRE)
It can be done regularly to look for any problems in the prostate area.
Imaging Tests means using machines to take pictures of the inside of the body.
More tests like MRIs or CT scans might be needed if there are worries that the
problem might come back.

Keeping Track of Repeat Occurrences
-Noticing Signs of Coming Back
-Increasing PSA level can mean that prostate cancer has come back.
-Symptoms: New pain, especially in the bones, losing weight for no clear
reason, or changes in how often you go to the bathroom or your stool.
-Handling Recurrence
-Local Recurrence: Might need extra treatments like radiation or surgery.
-Metastatic Recurrence: Treatments like hormone therapy, chemotherapy,
immunotherapy, or targeted therapy.
-Taking Care of Your Health for a Long Time

Healthy Lifestyle
Eat a mix of foods that includes fruits, vegetables, whole grains, and lean
meats.
Exercise means moving your body regularly to stay strong, keep your heart
healthy, and feel good overall.
- Weight Management: Keeping a healthy weight to lower the chances of
cancer coming back and to avoid other health problems.

Dealing with Side Effects
Incontinence: You can manage it with pelvic floor exercises, medicine, or
surgery.
Erectile Dysfunction: Medicines, tools, or therapy for sexual health.

Bone Health
Bone density checks: Regular tests to see how strong your bones are,
especially if you're using hormone therapy.
Supplements and Medicines: Calcium and vitamin D, plus medicines to make
bones stronger if necessary.

Heart Health
Checking: Regular visits to check blood pressure, cholesterol, and other heart
health risks.

Lifestyle: Eat heart-healthy foods and exercise to keep your heart healthy. Issues that affect how good life is.

Emotional and Psychological Support
Counseling: One-on-one or group help for dealing with anxiety, sadness, or other emotional problems.

Support Groups: Getting together with other people who have survived prostate cancer to help each other and share stories.

Sexual health and being close to someone.
Talk openly with your partner about any changes in sexual feelings and look for new ways to stay close and connected.
"Treatments and Therapies: Looking into ways to handle erectile dysfunction or other sexual health issues.

Managing Tiredness
- Save Energy: Mix activities with rest, decide what's important, and take things at a steady pace.
Exercise: Doing regular, moderate exercise can help reduce tiredness and increase your energy.

Health of the Bladder and Bowels
Pelvic Floor Exercises: Strengthening the muscles in your pelvic area to help you better control your bladder.
Diet changes: Taking care of bowel health by eating right and drinking plenty of water.

Fun and Social Events
Engagement: Keeping in touch with friends, family, and community events.
Hobbies: Doing things you enjoy to feel happy and have a purpose.

CHAPTER 9

DIET TO IMPROVE CANCER

Food is very important for helping the health of people with prostate cancer. There's no special diet that can cure prostate cancer, but making some food choices can help manage the condition, support treatment, and enhance overall well-being.

Here's a guide to a diet that is good for your prostate:

Key Dietary Recommendations

Fruits and vegetables are good for you because they have lots of vitamins, minerals, and fiber.

What to Eat:

Cruciferous vegetables like broccoli, cauliflower, Brussels sprouts, and kale have substances that might help slow down cancer.

Tomatoes: High in lycopene, which is an antioxidant that may reduce the risk of prostate cancer.

Berries like strawberries, blueberries, and raspberries are good for you because they have a lot of helpful nutrients called antioxidants.

Leafy greens like spinach, kale, and collard greens are packed with nutrients and help strengthen the immune system.

Healthy fats
This is important because treatments for prostate cancer can raise the chances of heart disease.

What to Eat:
Omega-3 fatty acids are found in fatty fish such as salmon, mackerel, and sardines, as well as in flaxseeds and chia seeds.
Olive Oil: Use it as a healthy cooking oil or in salad dressings.
Avocados: A food that has good fats for your heart.

Lean Proteins
Why: Protein is important for keeping muscles strong and healthy, especially when you are getting treatment.

What to Eat:
Fish: Full of omega-3 fats and protein.
Poultry: Chicken or turkey without skin for healthy protein.
Plant-Based Proteins: Beans, lentils, tofu, and tempeh are great sources of protein that don't have the unhealthy fats found in red meat.

Whole Grains
Why: Whole grains have a lot of fiber, which can help you control your weight and keep your digestion healthy.

What to Eat:
Oats: A great source of fiber and healthy nutrients.
Quinoa: A grain that has a lot of protein and is also high in fiber.
Brown rice has more vitamins and fiber than white rice.
Whole Wheat Foods: Bread, pasta, and cereals made from whole grains.

Eat less red and processed meats.
Why: Eating a lot of red and processed meats is connected to a greater chance of getting prostate cancer and other health problems.

What to Avoid:
Red Meat: Eat less beef, pork, and lamb.
Stay away from processed meats like bacon, sausages, and deli meats.

Milk and Calcium Consumption

Why: There are different opinions about how eating a lot of dairy affects the risk of prostate cancer, so it's a good idea to eat dairy in moderate amounts.

What to Eat:
Low-fat dairy products or plant-based options like almond or soy milk.
Enough Calcium; Try to have a good amount of calcium in your diet, but do not overdo it. You can find calcium in foods like leafy greens, almonds, and fortified products.

Drink enough water.
Why: Drinking enough water is important for your health and can help reduce problems from treatment, such as tiredness and a dry mouth.

What to Drink:
Like 8 to 10 glasses cup of water every day.
Herbal Teas: Try chamomile, green tea (just a little), or ginger tea for some different choices.
Limit Sweet Drinks: Stay away from soda and sugary drinks.

Foods to Eat for Certain Benefits
Foods High in Lycopene
Tomatoes, watermelon, and pink grapefruit contain lycopene, which is an antioxidant that may lower the chance of getting prostate cancer.

Soy Products
Tofu, tempeh, and soy milk have plant compounds that might help reduce PSA levels.

Green Tea
In moderation: Has catechins that might help slow down the growth of prostate cancer.

Pomegranate Juice
Antioxidants: Some research shows that pomegranate juice might help slow down the growth of prostate cancer.

Lifestyle Considerations
Portion Control: Stay at a healthy weight by eating balanced meals with the right amount of food.
Stay Active: Eat healthy foods and exercise regularly to control your weight and stay healthy.

- Limit Alcohol: If you drink, do it in moderation because too much alcohol can affect your treatment and health.

CHAPTER 10

HELP AND RESOURCES

Dealing with prostate cancer can be hard, but there are many resources and support options to help you. Here's a summary of groups, websites, support for patients, and money-help programs that can offer assistance.

Groups and Charities
American Cancer Society (ACS)
Provides help, information, and resources for cancer patients and their families.

Website: org
Prostate Cancer Foundation (PCF) is an organization focused on fighting prostate cancer.
Concentrates on giving money for research and offering learning materials.
Website: pcf.org

ZERO - The End of Prostate Cancer
Helps patients by giving support, teaching, and speaking up for awareness and research about prostate cancer.
Website: zerocancer.org

Men's Health Network
Offers information about men's health problems, like prostate cancer, and encourages awareness and support.
Website: menshealthnetwork.org

Online Resources:

Cancer Treatment
Offers free help, such as counseling, support groups, and learning workshops.
Website: cancercare.org

National Cancer Institute (NCI)
Provides complete information about prostate cancer, treatment choices, clinical studies, and research.

MedlinePlus.
A service from the National Library of Medicine that offers trustworthy information about prostate cancer and related subjects.
Website: medlineplus.gov

HealthUnlocked Prostate Cancer Group
An online group where patients and their caregivers can talk about their experiences and help each other.
Website: healthunlocked.com/prostate-cancer

Cancer Help Group
Provides online support groups, helpful information, and health programs for cancer patients and their families.
Website: cancersupportcommunity.org

Helping Patients Speak Up
Prostate Cancer Supporters

People or groups focused on educating others, shaping rules, and helping with research and care for prostate cancer.

Patient Advocate Foundation is a group that helps patients with their healthcare needs and problems.
Offers support and financial help to patients with serious and long-lasting illnesses.
Website: patientadvocate.org

Programs to help support and advocate for people with prostate cancer.
Many groups provide training and chances for patients to participate in laws
and policy efforts.

Money Help Programs
Cancer Financial Help Group (CFAC)
A group of organizations that assist cancer patients with their money problems.
Website: cancerfac.org

HealthWell Foundation
Helps pay for medicine and treatment costs that you have to pay yourself.
Website: healthwellfoundation.org

Patient Access Network Foundation (PAN) is an organization that helps people
get access to the medical care and treatments they need.
Provides money to help patients who don't have enough insurance pay for
their treatment costs.
Website: panfoundation.org

Co-Pay Help Program
Helps patients who have insurance and meet certain financial and health
requirements with co-payments, insurance costs, and deductibles.
Website: copays.org

NeedyMeds is a resource that helps people find assistance for medical costs
and medications.
A place to help you find programs that can help pay for medicine and
healthcare.

CHAPTER 11

CONCLUSION

Overall Summary on Prostate Cancer
Prostate cancer is a common type of cancer in men, especially older men. Although it can be a dangerous and serious illness, new ways to find, treat, and manage it have greatly helped many patients do better.

Finding prostate cancer early is very important for treating it well. Getting regular tests, like PSA tests and digital rectal exams, can help catch the disease early when it's easier to treat. Knowing the risks, like age, family background, and lifestyle choices, can help in spotting problems early and preventing them.

There are different ways to treat prostate cancer. These include watching it closely, surgery, radiation, hormone treatment, chemotherapy, immunotherapy, and targeted treatments. The type of treatment depends on how advanced the cancer is, how serious it is, the patient's overall health, and what the patient wants. Each treatment can have different side effects that may affect physical health, feelings, and sexual health. Dealing with these side effects is an important part of the treatment.

Dealing with prostate cancer needs both medical care and help for feelings and mental health. Creating a good support network, choosing healthy habits, and getting help with money and feelings can assist patients and their families in dealing with the difficulties of the illness.

In general, prostate cancer can be handled well, especially if found early. Thanks to continuous research and progress in medical science, things are getting better for prostate cancer patients. By keeping up with information, living healthily, and getting the right treatment and help, people with prostate cancer can live happy lives.

www.ingramcontent.com/pod-product-compliance
Lightning Source LLC
Chambersburg PA
CBHW051712250726
48653CB00007B/2983